Reiki Friends®
The Adventure Begins

Written by Ruby Reiki Studio

How to say these words:

Reiki: Ray-Key

Sensei: Sen-Say

Usui: You-Sue-E

Takata: Tah-Kah-Tah

A big storm was coming.

Long before the people of Japan knew the storm was coming the bears knew. The bears forgot about their daily routine of playing in the woods, hunting for food, and enjoying the sun. They needed to find shelter. They set out to look for a safe place until after the storm passed.

They looked all over for a safe place. The old hollow tree was too small for all of them to hide in. The big rock by the river was sure to flood. They needed to find a safe and dry place to stay out of the storm.

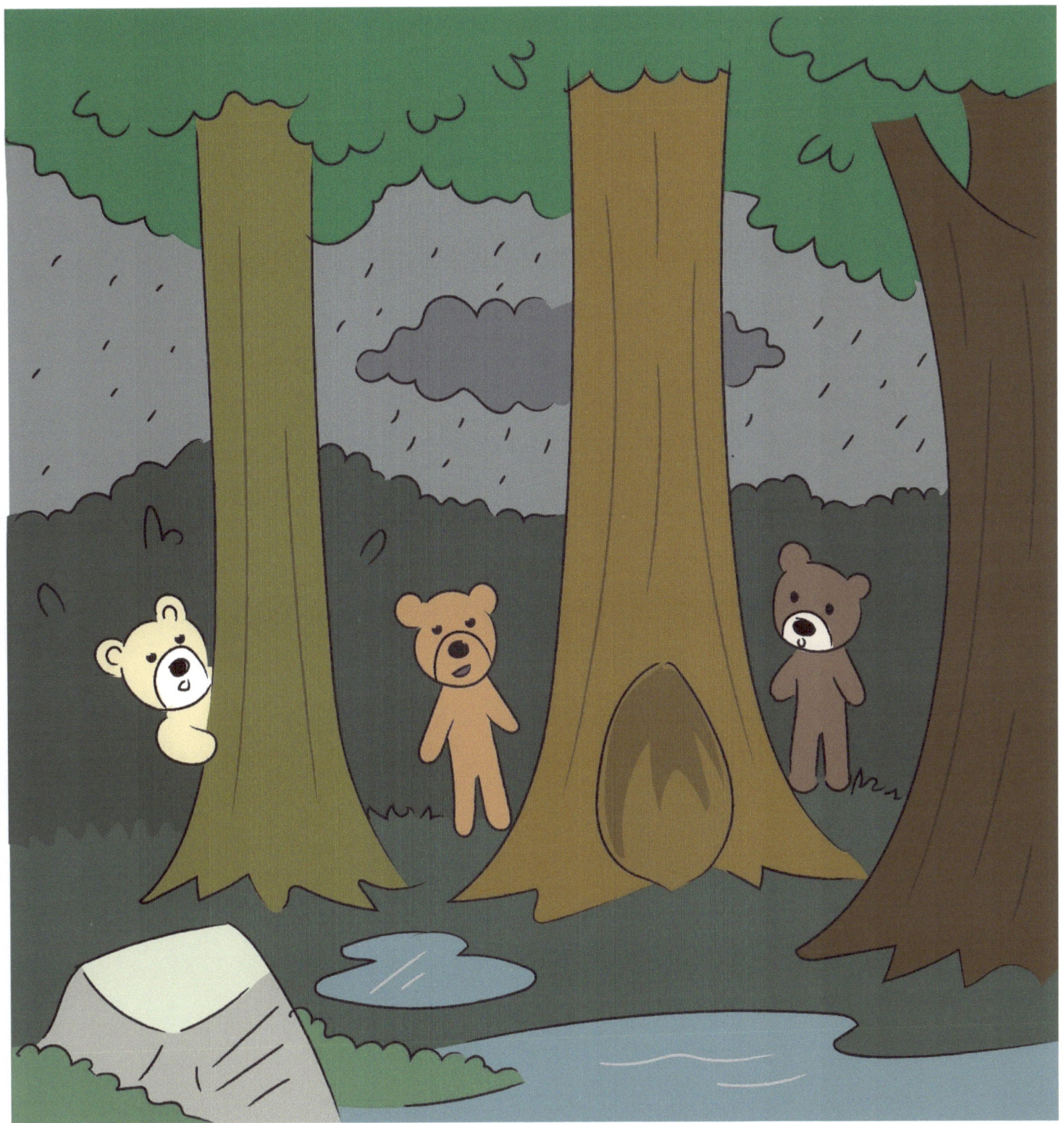

They found a cave and carefully entered the dark and scary place. The little bear wished there were at least some fireflies that he often saw in the woods around to light the way.

Soon there was a glow up ahead in the cave. The bears moved closer to the light. Instead of fireflies they found a man sitting in front of a nice warm and bright fire. He was sitting with his legs under him and it looked like he was sleeping. The bears moved closer. Suddenly the man's eyes opened and the bears froze in their tracks.

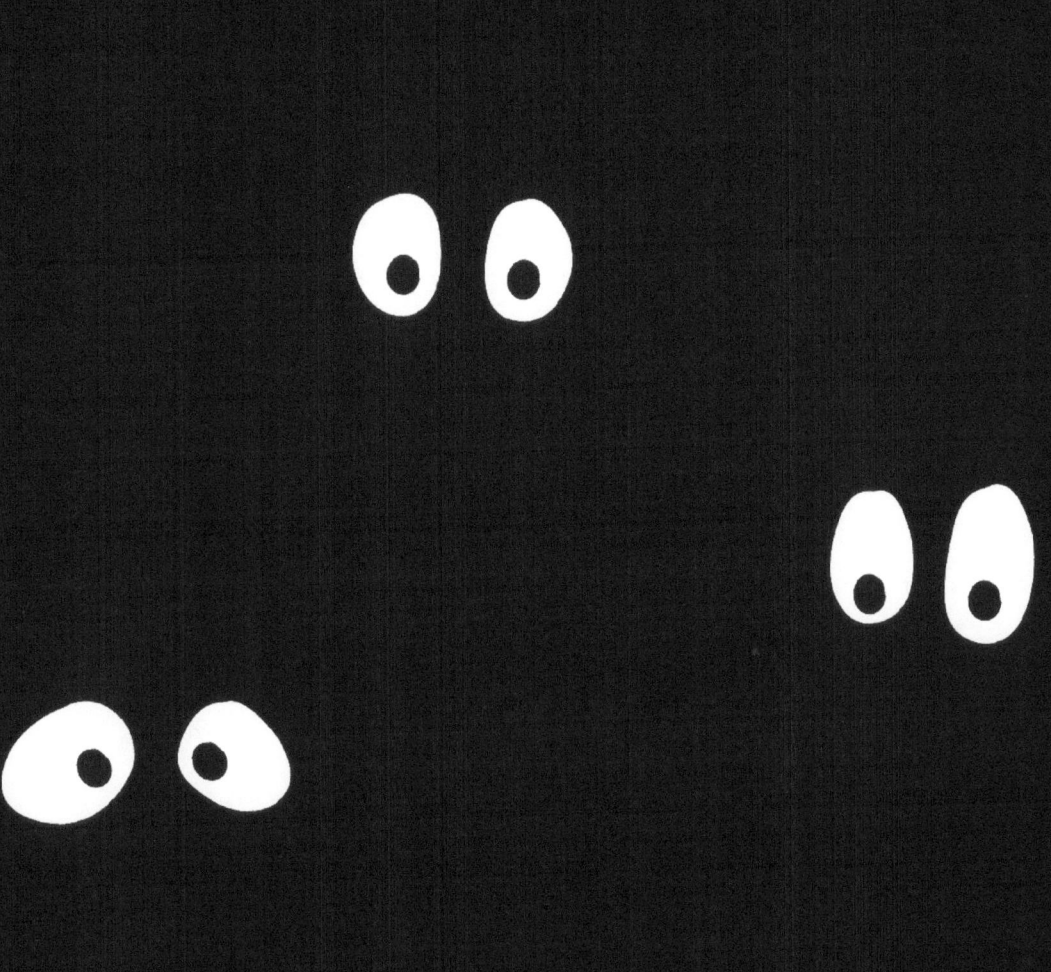

Usui Sensei then told the bears that he was not sleeping when they found him. He told them he was meditating and explained that was a way to focus his thoughts. He explained to the bears about something he called Reiki. He explained that it was a special way to make people feel better.

Sensei told the bears that he was going to give the animals the power to do Reiki so that they could go out into the world and help others.

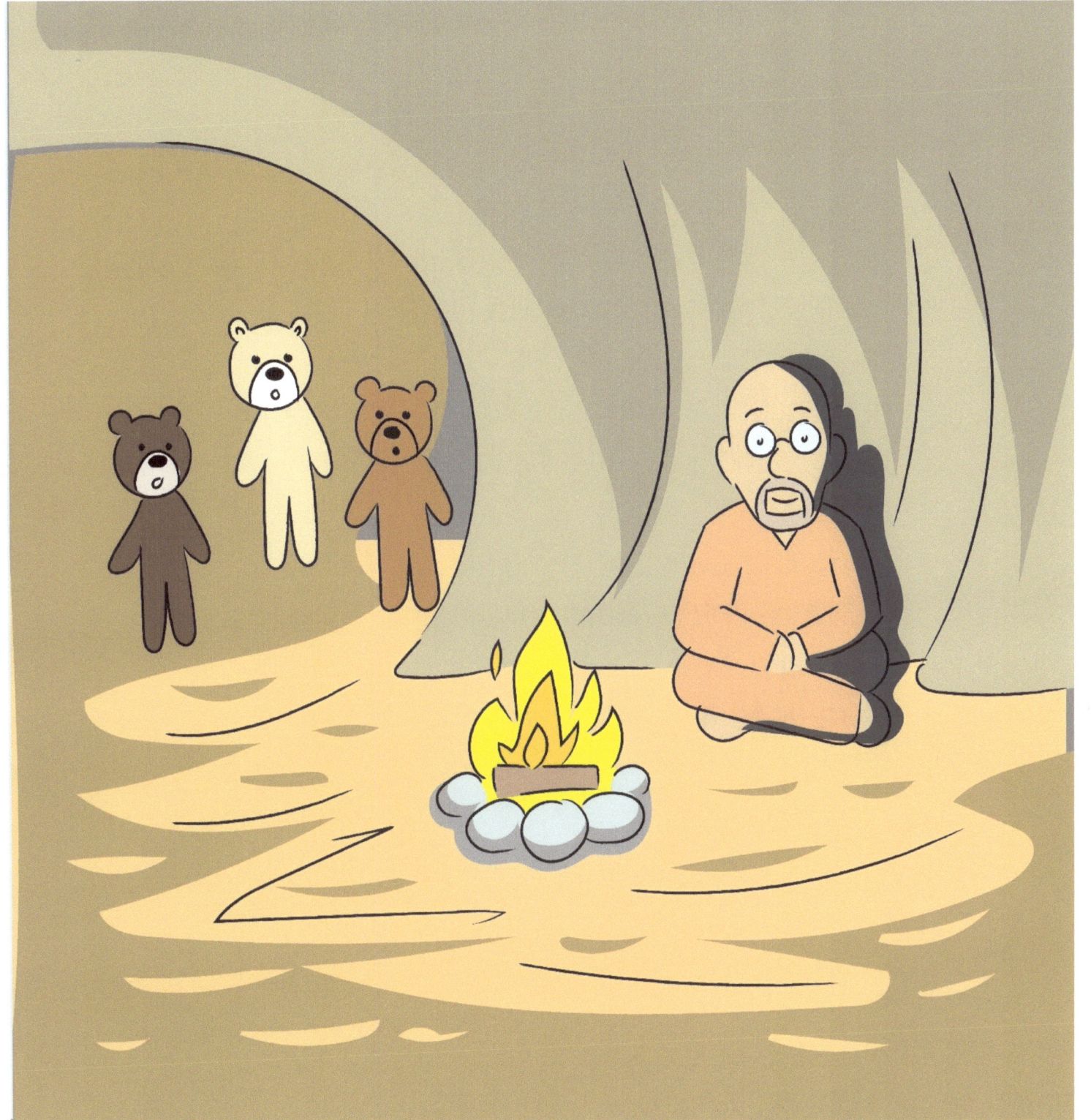

They sat around the warm fire and listened to the soothing voice of Usui Sensei. He explained that Reiki is a special energy that relaxes and helps heal living creatures.

Sensei gave the bears the power to use the loving energy of Reiki to help and heal all living creatures. The bears were told they were to go to America to spread their new gift of Reiki.

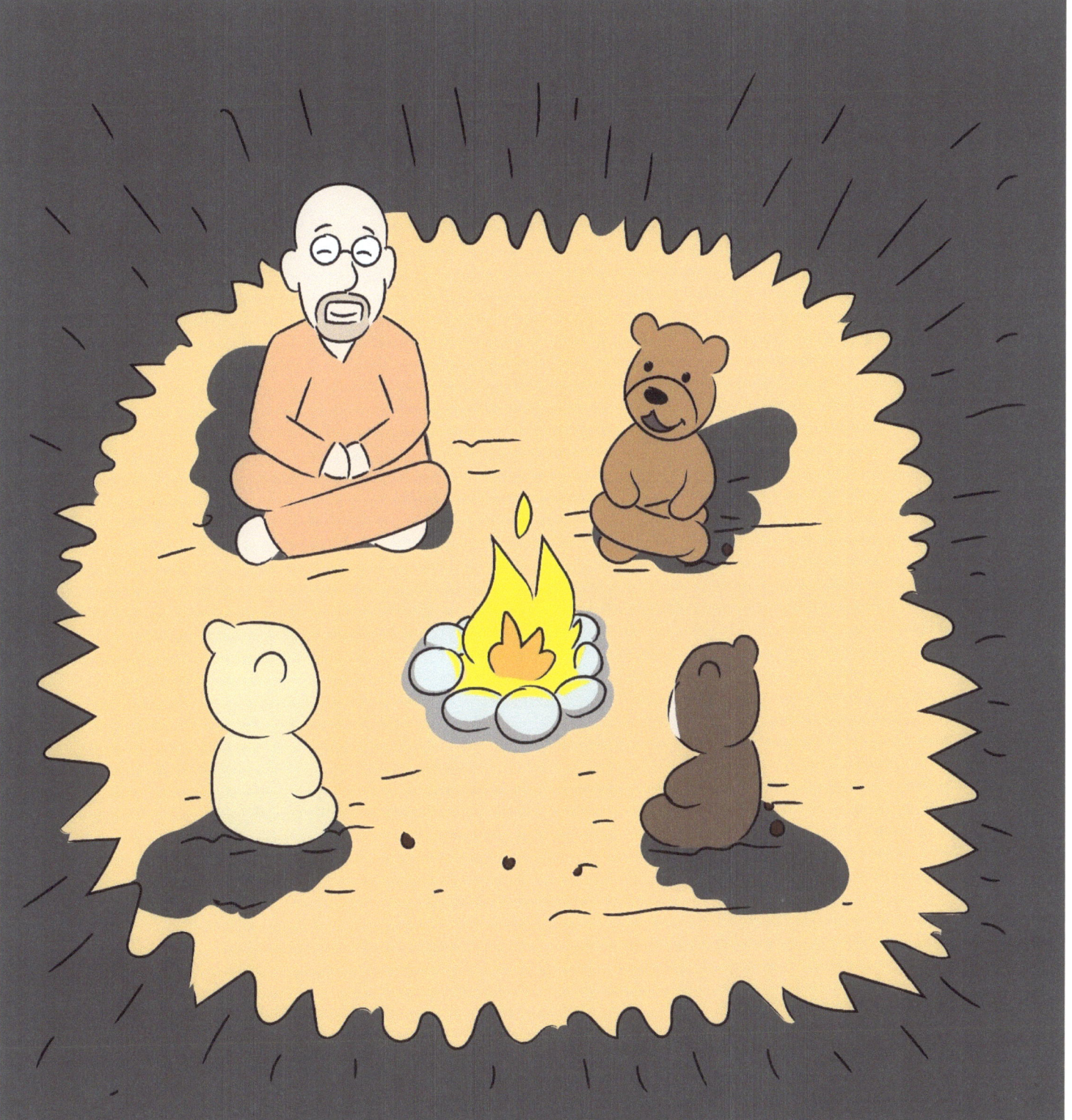

The bears boarded a ship headed towards America. A short time into the trip the sky turned gray and the wind began to howl. Waves started to rock the boat and many of the sailors started to get seasick.

The bears remembered what Sensei taught them. They used their Reiki on the sailors to help calm their flippty floppity tummies. The bears placed their paws on the sailors and allowed the Reiki energy to help calm the sailors.

The storm ended and the sea was calm again. The rest of the trip was quiet and the bears got some much needed sleep.

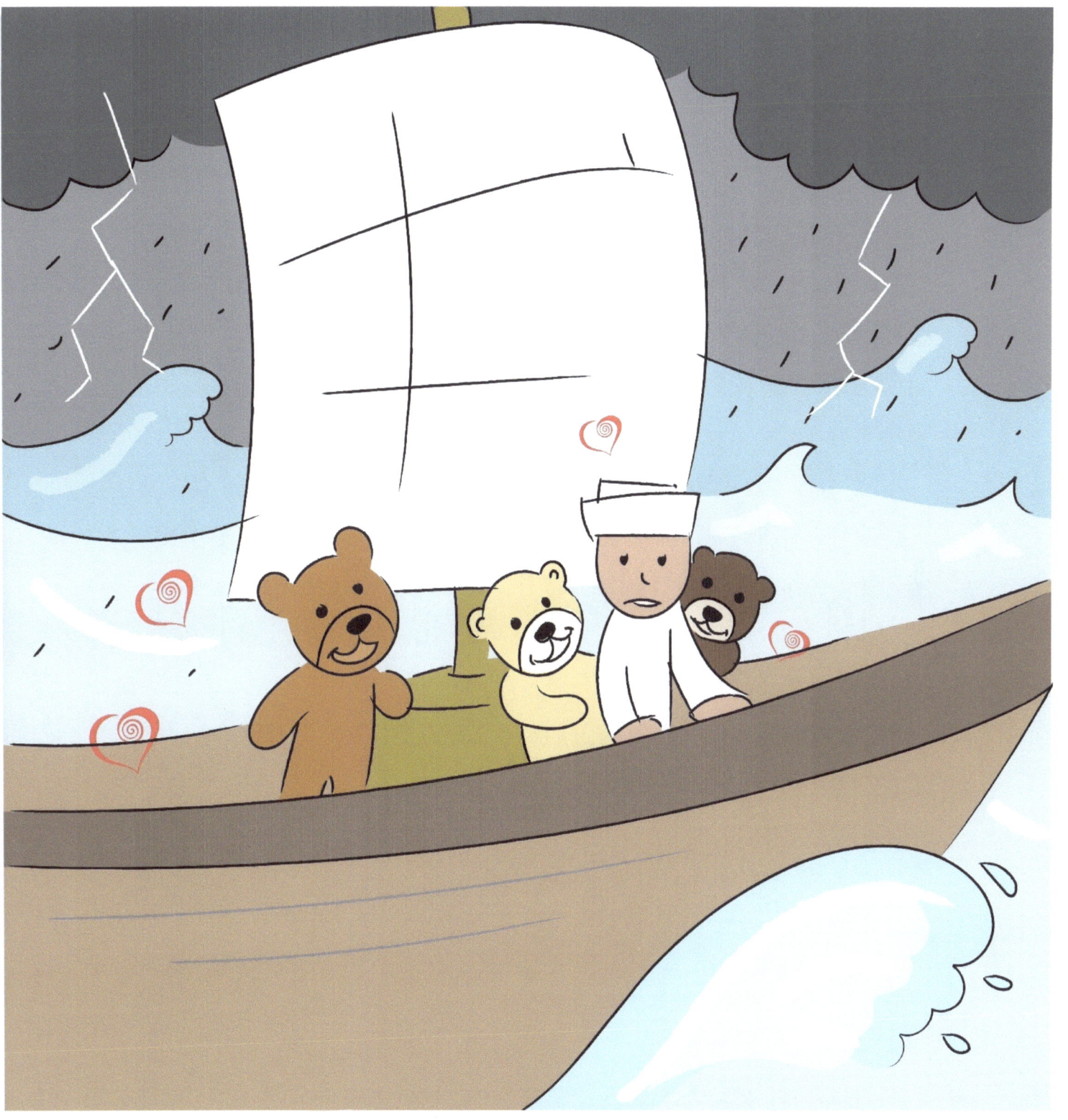

In the morning the ship docked in the beautiful island of Hawaii. The bears decided to get off the ship. On the island, the bears met a woman named Mrs. Takata that also knew about Reiki.

Mrs. Takata invited the bears back to her house for a yummy lunch. Mrs. Takata spent hours teaching the bears what she knew about Reiki and how they could help others just by placing their paws on them.

The bears were even more excited about helping others using Reiki. Mrs. Takata let her dog join the bears on their trip.

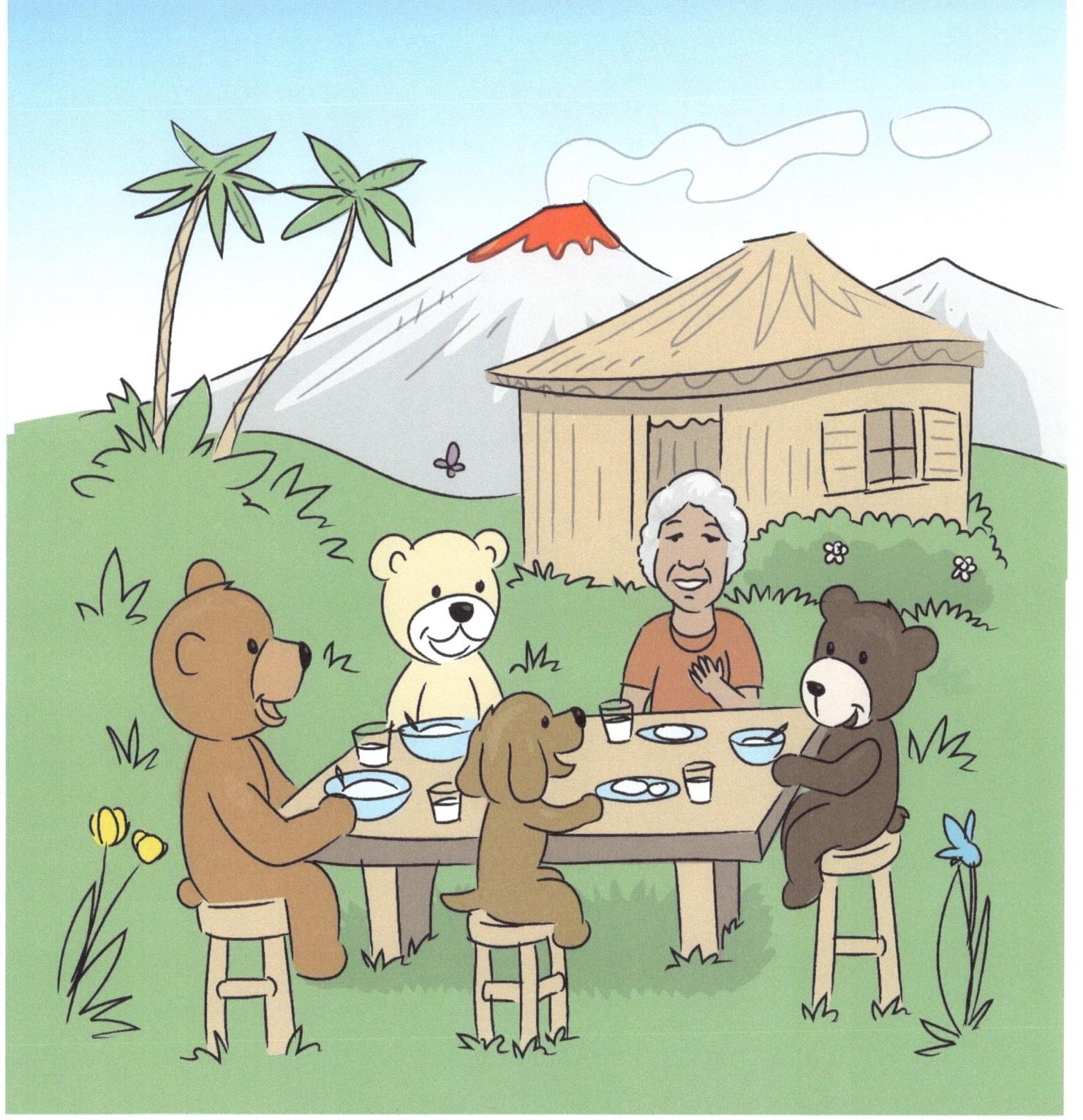

The animals boarded a big cruise ship and headed towards California.

There were many people who had flippity floppity tummies just like the first ship. The animals held their paws against the people and used Reiki to help the people feel better.

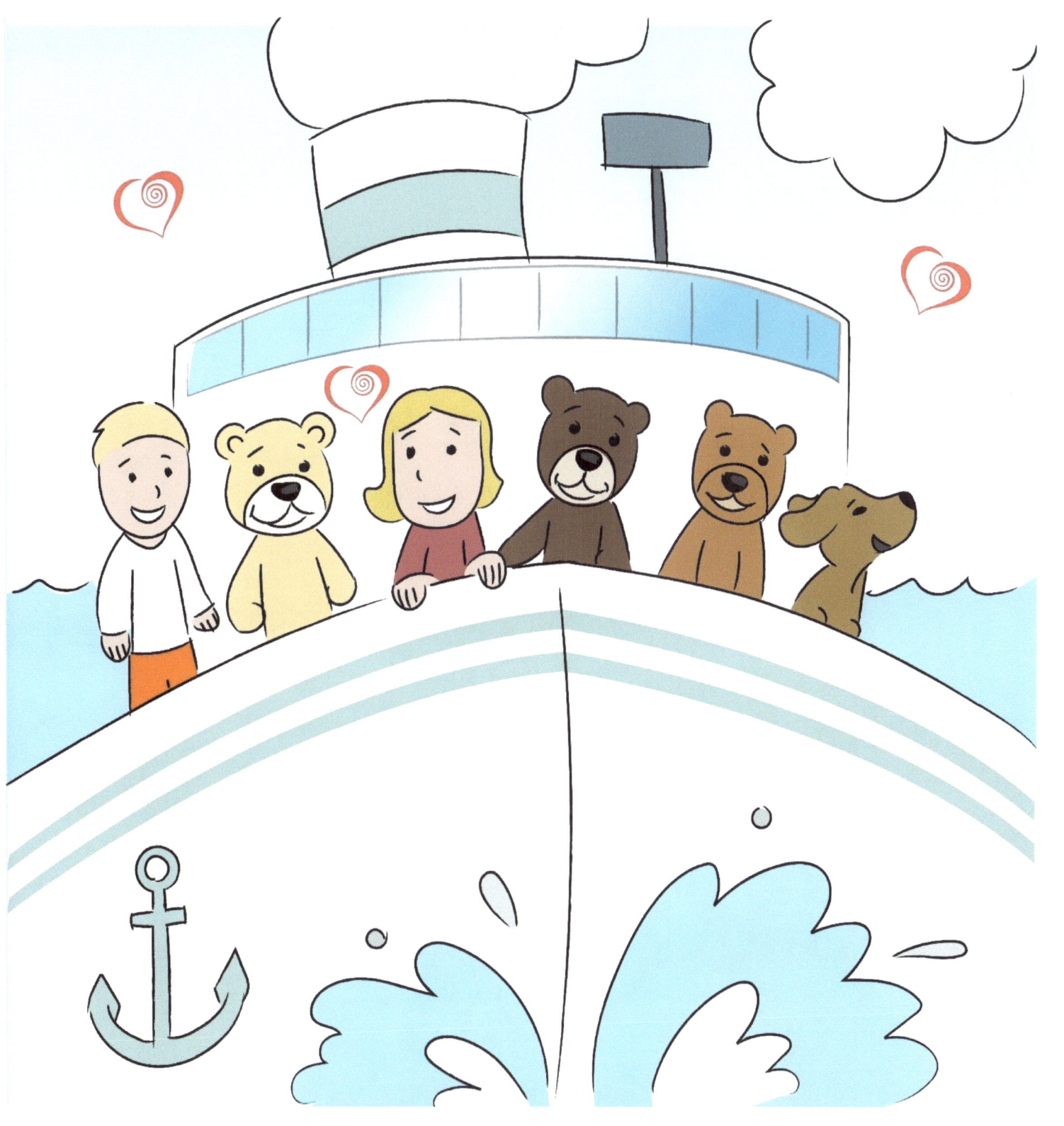

Their first stop in America was a children's hospital. The animals found all kinds of children that did not feel well. Some were very sick. All of the children were happy to see the friendly animals.

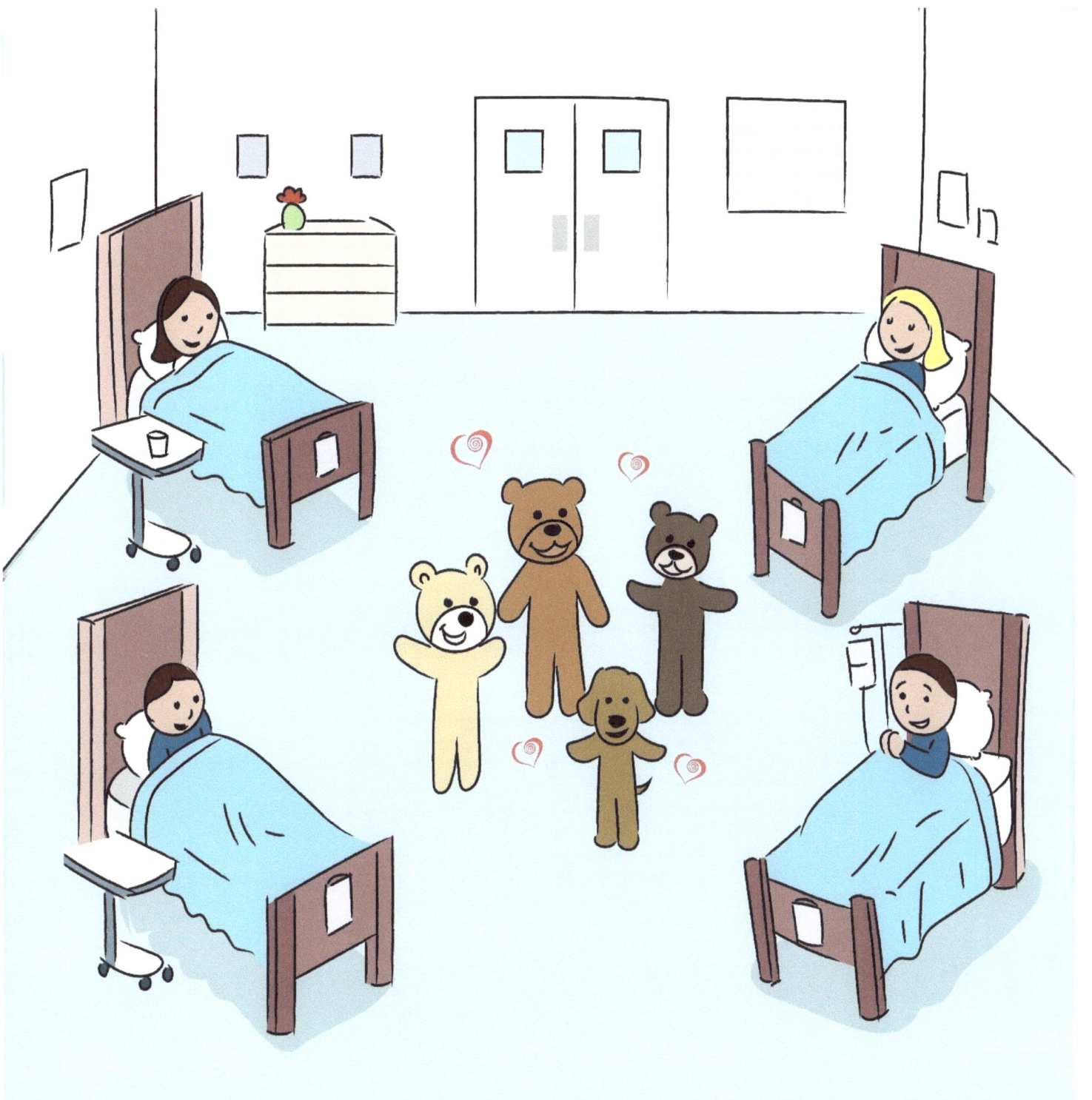

The animals were quick to snuggle up to the children and use Reiki on them.

Many of the children started to feel better as the animals held them.

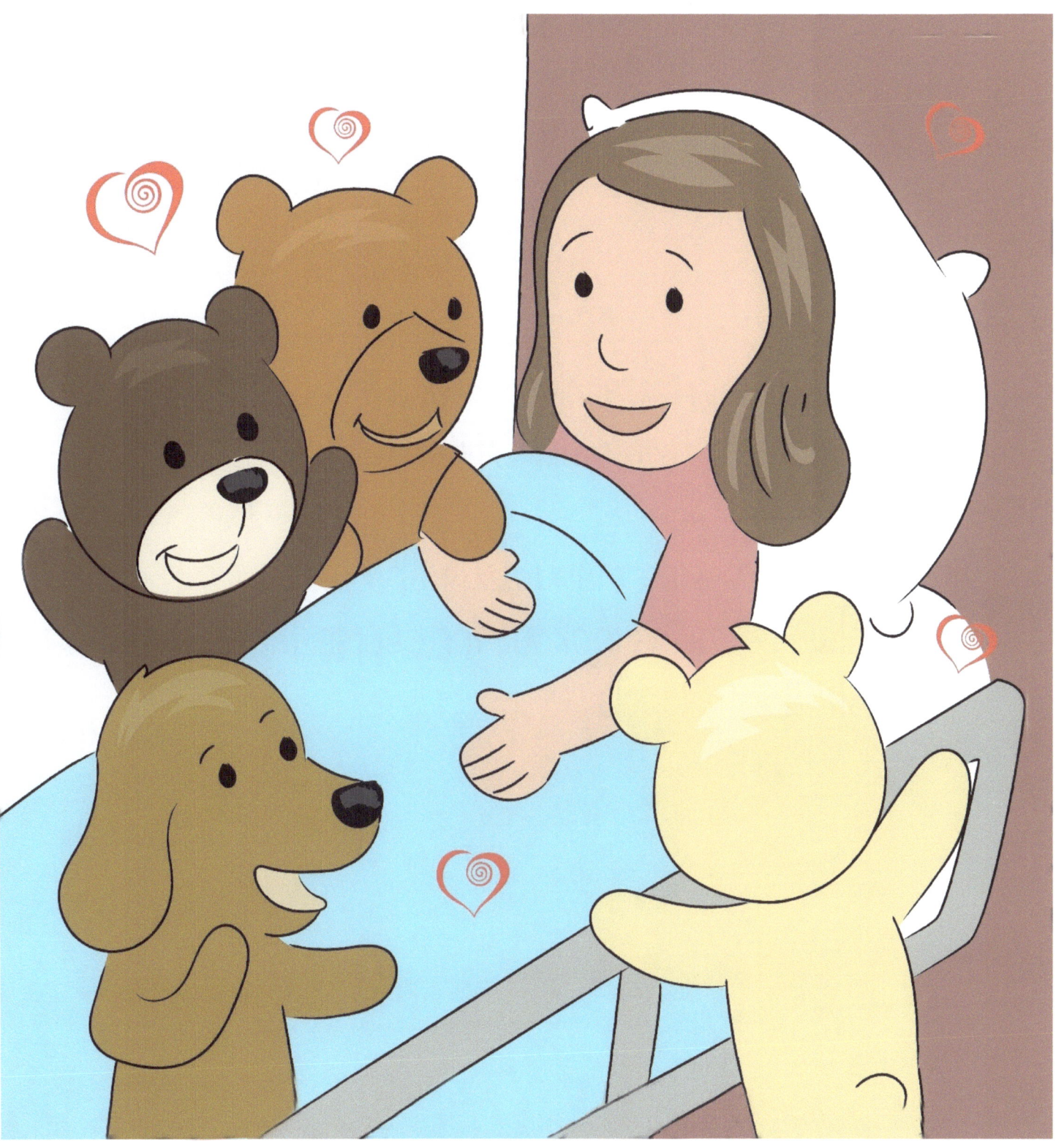

The animals traveled across the country looking to help others with Reiki.

They traveled many days and nights always on the lookout for people that did not feel well.

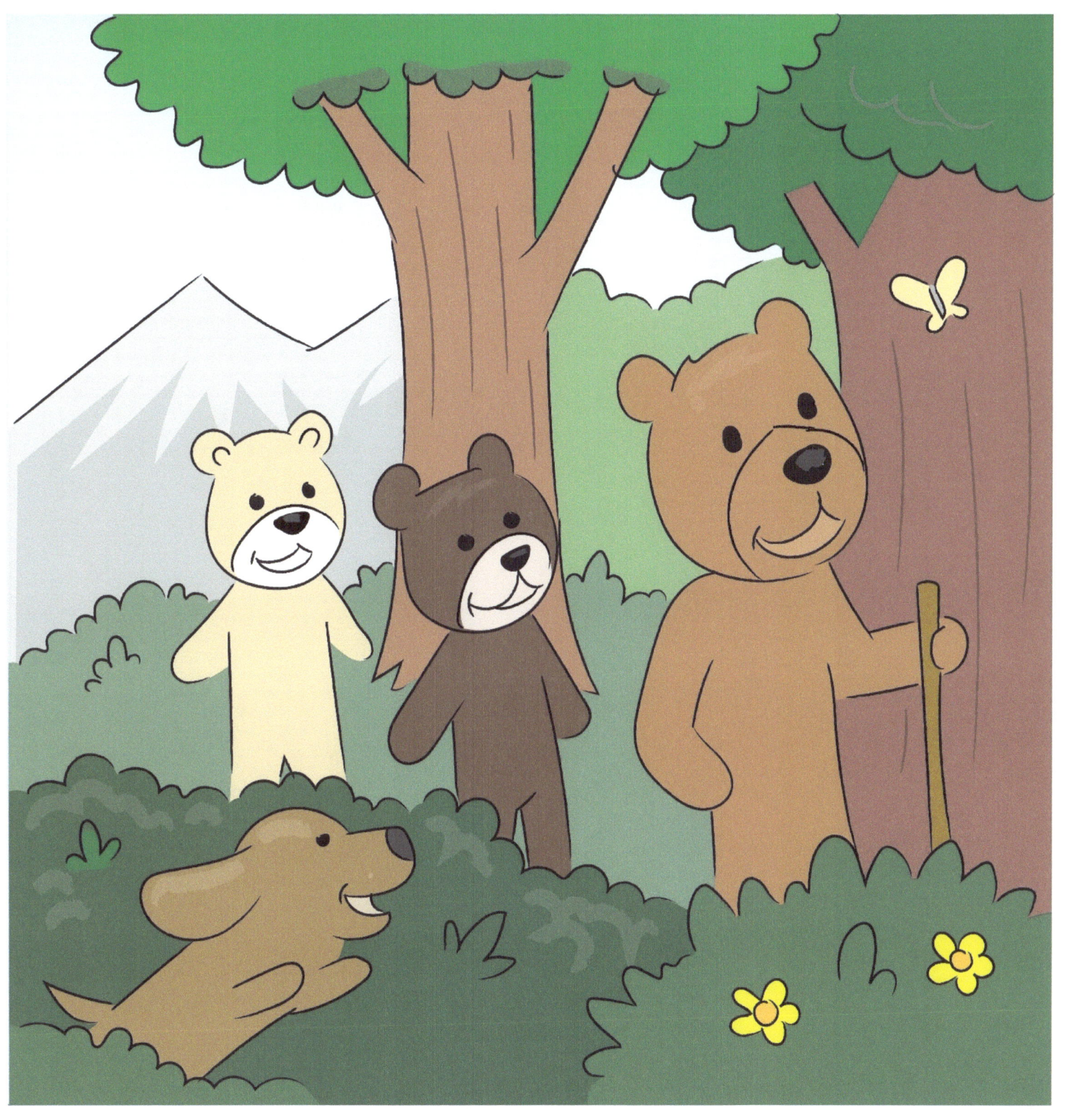

They stopped at a zoo where they made friends with a monkey and giraffe that wanted to learn Reiki and join them on their trip.

The animals asked the zookeeper for permission and the zookeeper let them go so they could help children.

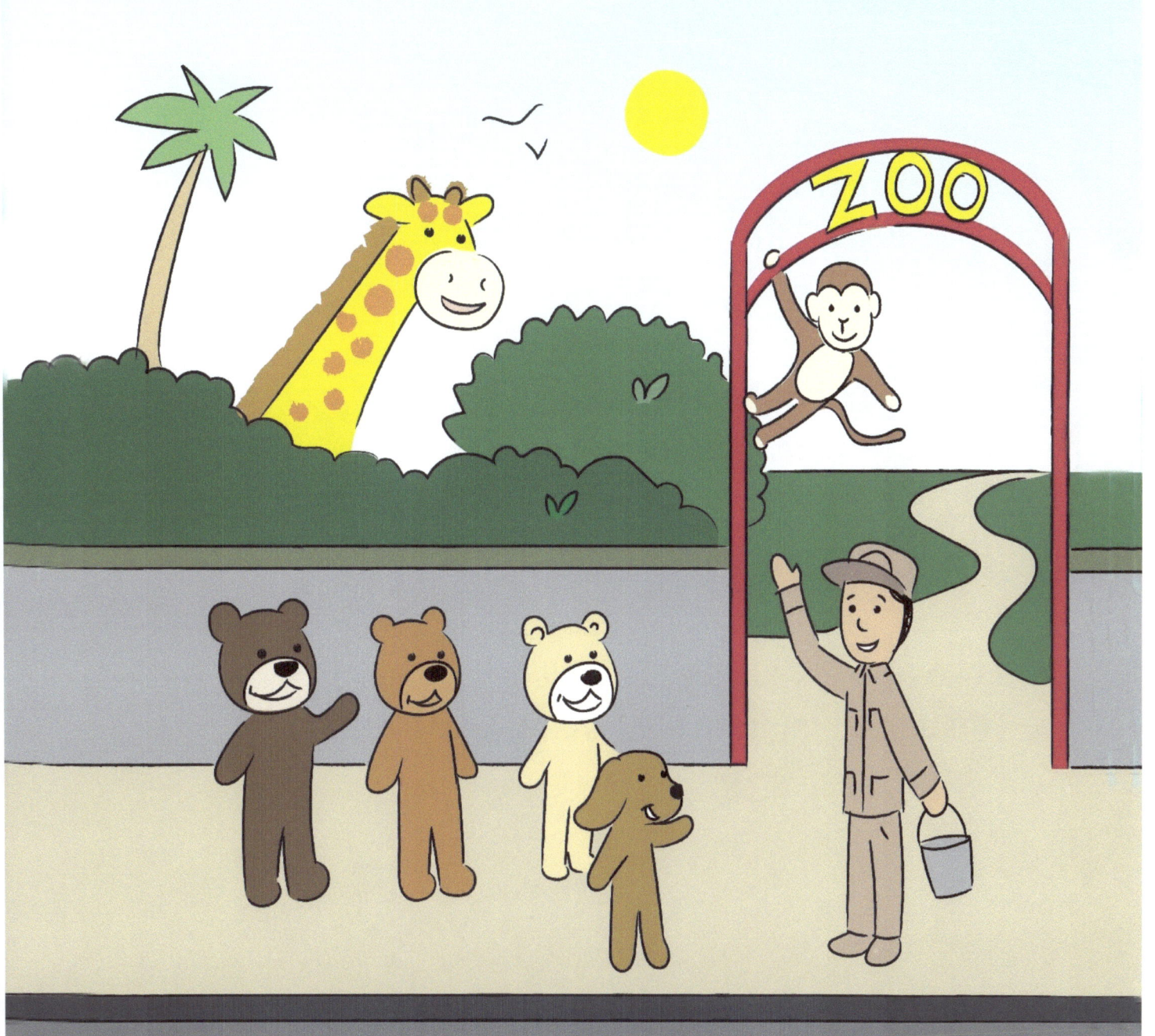

The animals met lots of people that needed help to feel better.

They met a farmer that had a bad headache. The animals helped the farmer feel better by using Reiki. The farmer was so happy that he allowed his cow to join the animals on their journey.

The animals taught the cow how to use Reiki and continued on their way with their new friend.

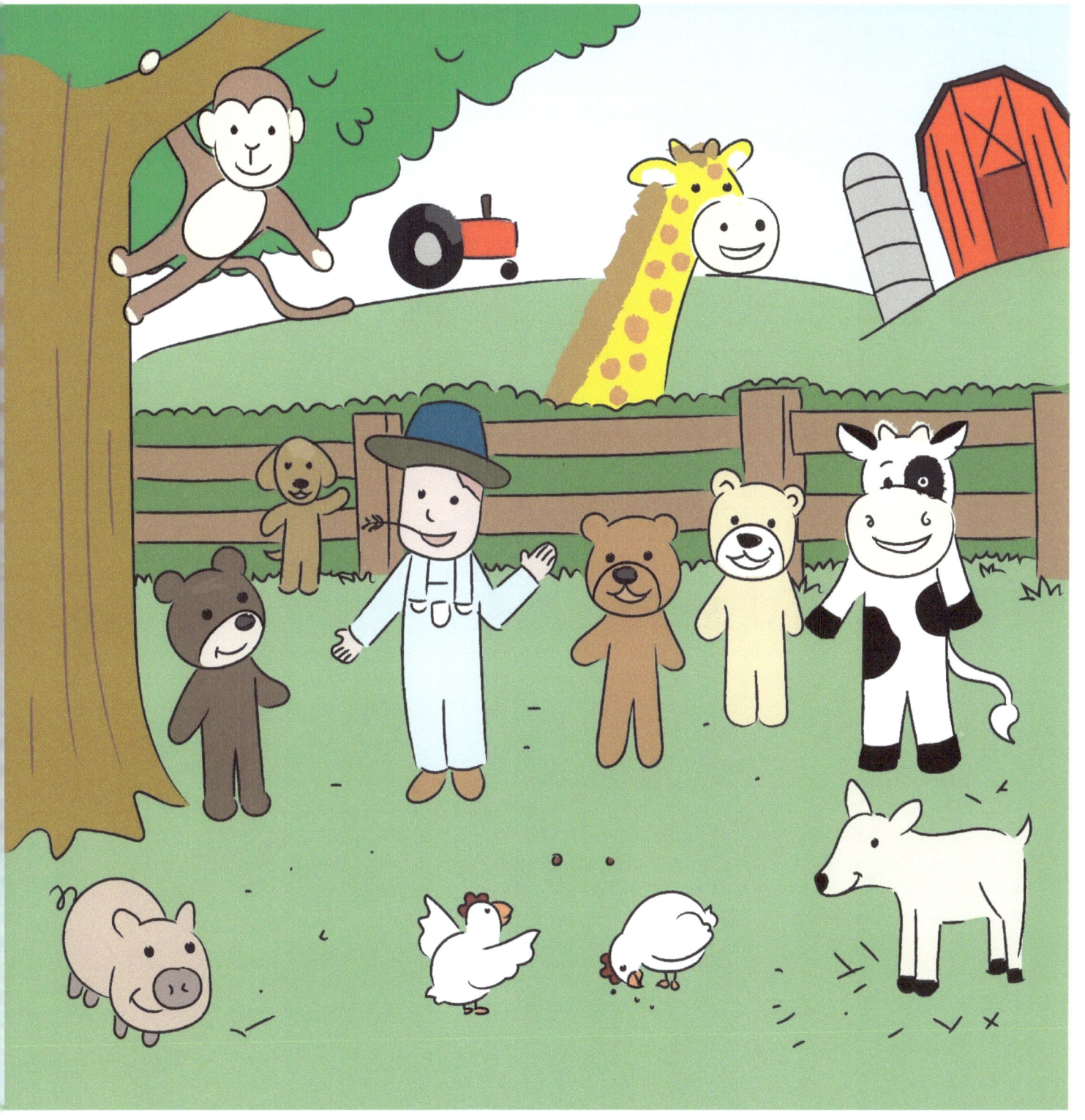

The animals finally reached the Ruby Reiki Studio where they were welcomed by Ruby. Ruby also knew about Reiki. Together, the animals and Ruby made a plan to get the animals where they were needed anywhere in the world.

Ruby introduced them to ReiKi ReNew, a special system for sending daily Reiki energy to the Ruby Reiki Studio heart logo.

The animals had become such good friends that they decided that they wanted to be called the Reiki Friends. Ruby gave them all special T-shirts or collars with their new name and her special heart logo on them.

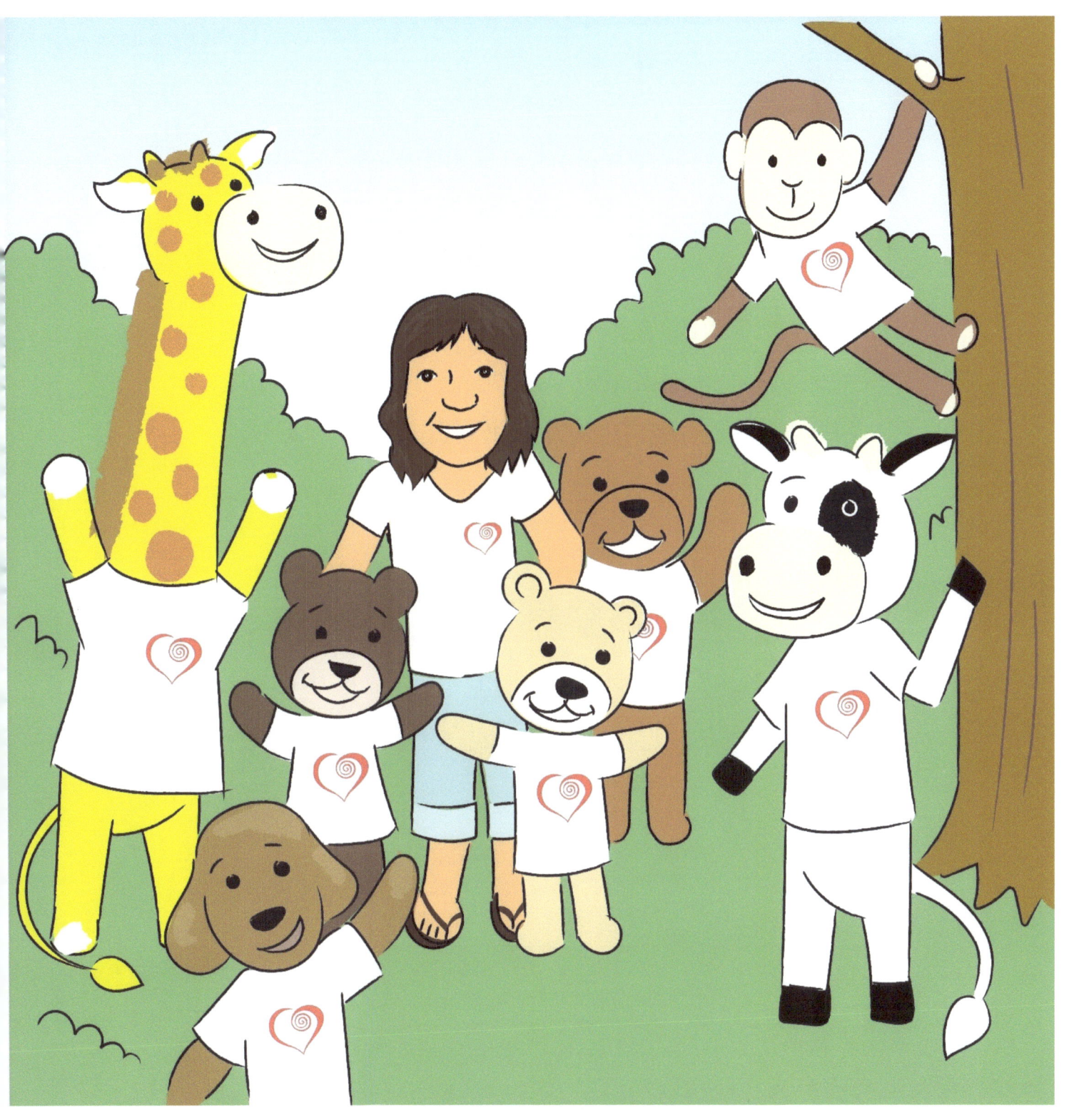

Reiki Friends receive loving Reiki energy every single day through the special logo and they share that special energy with anyone that holds them.

Reiki Friends wait to be sent to their new home where they will happily snuggle with children of all ages. They radiate loving, healing, relaxing Reiki energy to all that need it.

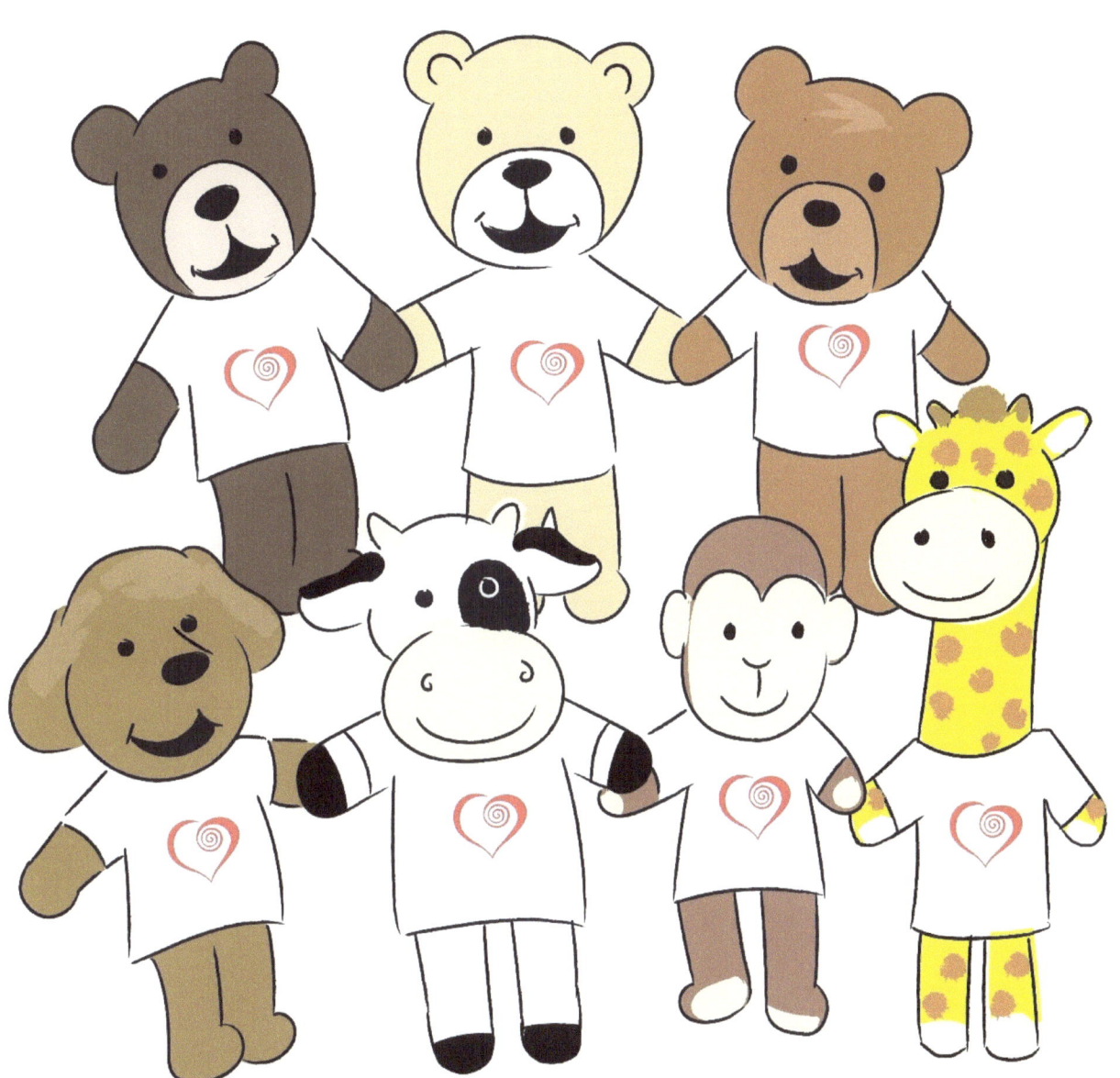

For more information and to get your own Reiki Friend
Go to www.ReikiFriends.net